Bread Machine Cookbook For Beginners

The Ultimate Guide To Easy-To-Follow Bread Machine Recipes To Cook For Fun With Your Family And Friends

Giulia Baker

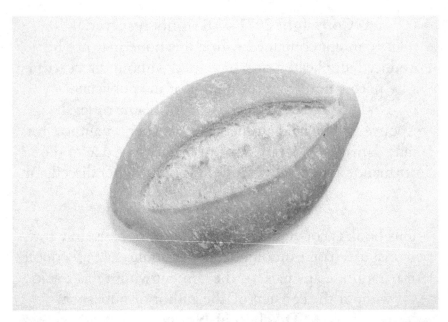

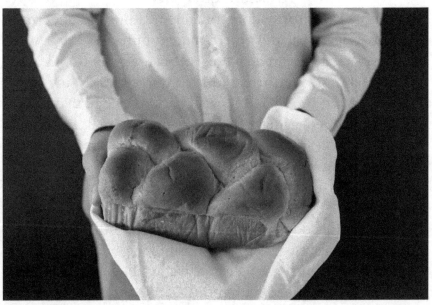

Table of Contents

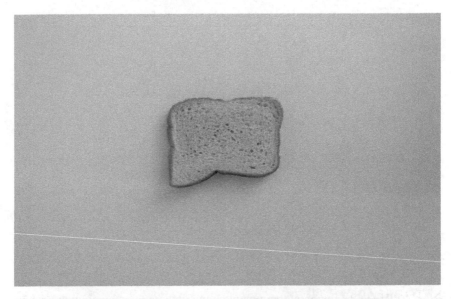

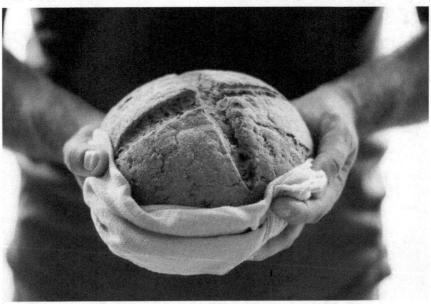

Introduction

Since then we all love bread, before we discover fire, it has been on the menu and we enjoy it so much. But as time goes by, we replace fire and primitive cooking methods with bread machine, from traditional baking to modern baking.

Modern baking using bread machines are more conventional to people who are always on the go. They are also invented to make baking more a lot easier. Considering what type of bread machine to consider will be depending on the volume you always you make. Time to time there will always be new technologies on bread machine but they all give you positive result- yummy bread.

Healthy and tasty bread surely is made from the best quality ingredients. Not only the freshest things that you can put in the mixing bowl, but the right cooking process also determine the delicacy and the safety of the bread.

Basically, bread is made from flour, water, yeast, and salt. After measuring the ingredients according to the recipe, the second step of making bread is mixing the ingredients. This step can be done using a mixer or manually kneading by hands. No matter what tool do you use, the dough should reach the right consistency. After the dough reaches the right consistency, the dough will be left to sit for a period of time to allow the fermentation process. Once it rises to double its size, it should be punched to expel the air inside the dough. Next, it is time to divide and fill the dough according to the baker's desire. After that, the filled dough should be sat for the final fermentation and later, bake the bread.

Well, making bread seems to be a long way to go. There are many steps to take in order to get soft and yummy bread. The right consistency of the dough is the first main key to generate perfect bread. However, this step is slightly tricky, and often makes people fail in making bread. One way to check the right consistency is by stretching a little bit of the dough. If the dough is stretched, it will become wide, transparent, and will not rip. If the dough doesn't reach the proper consistency, hard bread will certainly be resulted.

Luckily, a bread machine comes to be the best partner for every amateur baker who wants to bake bread from home. As a true assistant, the bread machine not only shortens the steps of making bread, but it also makes the process a lot easier. You just need to put the ingredients inside the baking tin, cover the bread machine, and hit the buttons. The bread machine ensures you to get the perfect bread that is usually found in famous bakeries. The great thing about this appliance is that the bread machine does all the bread making process for you, unattended. While you are waiting for the bread machine do its job, you still can do all your daily activities or enjoy your favorite movie.

Making bread seemed to be so impossible that most people never dreamed of doing so. However, a bread machine changes it all. Now, millions of people turn their lovely kitchen to bakeries. Everyone can enjoy the freshest, healthiest, and tastiest bread from their own warm kitchen without spending too much money for it.

The most beneficial of having a bread machine is having fresh bread at the tip of your finger. You just need to prepare the necessary ingredients ahead of time, and let the machine do the work.

Secondly, you can control the ingredients, add delicious ingredients that suits to your palate.

Bread machines make more than bread. Bread machine is not just for making breads; you can use it to make jam, pasta and dough for your homemade pizza.

Superior taste and quality of bread, they are easy to operate. So you don't have to worry whether you are a good baker or not. Bread machines are programmed to make perfect heavenly breads. Same process in traditional making of bread you must also consider following instructions and considering that you are using a machine the right settings in cooking bread. Baking using bread machine will also bring out one's creativity.

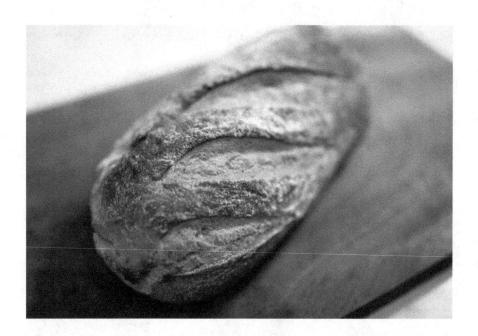

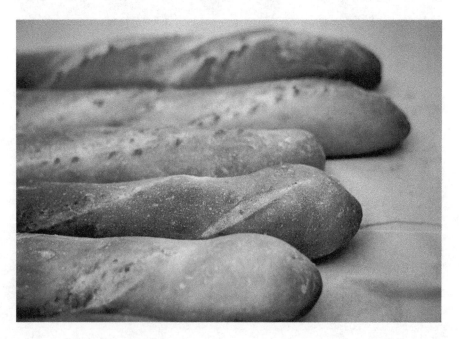

Basic Breads

1. Anadama Bread

Preparation Time: 3 hours

Cooking Time: 45 minutes

Servings: 2 loaves

Ingredients:

1/2 cup sunflower seeds

2 teaspoon bread machine yeast

4 1/2 cups bread flour

3/4 cup yellow cornmeal

2 tablespoon unsalted butter, cubed

1 1/2 teaspoon salt

1/4 cup dry skim milk powder

1/4 cup molasses

1 1/2 cups water, with a temperature of 80 to 90 degrees F (26 to 32 degrees C)

Directions:

Put all the ingredients in the pan, except the sunflower seeds, in this order: water, molasses, milk, salt, butter, cornmeal, flour, and yeast.

Place the pan in the machine and close the lid.

Put the sunflower seeds in the fruit and nut dispenser.

Turn the machine on and choose the basic setting and your desired color of the crust. Press start.

Nutrition:

Calories: 130 calories;

Total Carbohydrate: 25 g

Total Fat: 2 g

Protein: 3 g

2. Apricot Oat

Preparation Time: 1 hour 25 minutes

Cooking Time: 25 minutes

Servings: 1 loaf

Ingredients:

4 1/4 cups bread flour

2/3 cup rolled oats

1 tablespoon white sugar

2 teaspoons active dry yeast

1 1/2 teaspoons salt

1 teaspoon ground cinnamon

2 tablespoons butter, cut up

1 2/3 cups orange juice

1/2 cup diced dried apricots

2 tablespoons honey, warmed

Directions:

Into the pan of bread machine, put the bread ingredients in the order suggested by manufacturer. Then pout in dried apricots before the knead cycle completes.

Immediately remove bread from machine when it's done and then glaze with warmed honey. Let to cool completely prior to serving.

Nutrition:

Calories: 80 calories;

Total Carbohydrate: 14.4 g

Cholesterol: 5 mg

Total Fat: 2.3 g

Protein: 1.3 g

Sodium: 306 mg

Spice and Herb Breads

3. Cumin Bread

Preparation Time: 3 hours 30 minutes

Cooking Time: 15 minutes

Servings: 8

Ingredients:

5 1/3 cups bread machine flour, sifted

1½ teaspoon kosher salt

1½ Tablespoon sugar

1 Tablespoon bread machine yeast

1¾ cups lukewarm water

2 Tablespoon black cumin

3 Tablespoon sunflower oil

Directions:

Place all the dry and liquid ingredients in the pan and follow the instructions for your bread machine.

Set the baking program to BASIC and the crust type to MEDIUM.

If the dough is too dense or too wet, adjust the amount of flour and liquid in the recipe.

When the program has ended, take the pan out of the bread machine and let cool for 5 minutes.

Shake the loaf out of the pan. If necessary, use a spatula.

Wrap the bread with a kitchen towel and set it aside for an hour. Otherwise, you can cool it on a wire rack.

Nutrition:

Calories: 368 calories;Total Carbohydrate: 67.1 g

Cholesterol: 0 mg Total Fat: 6.5 g Protein: 9.5 g

Sodium: 444 mg Sugar: 2.5 g

Grain, Seed and Nut Bread

4. Oat Bread

Preparation Time: 1 hour 30 minutes

Cooking Time: 40 minutes

Servings: 2-3 loaves

Ingredients:

1 cup Oats

1⅜ to 1½ cups Water

2 tablespoons Butter or margarine

¼ cup Honey

2 teaspoons Salt

3 cups Bread flour red star brand

2½ teaspoons Active dry yeast

Directions:

Place all Ingredients in bread pan, using the least amount of liquid listed in the recipe. Select medium crust setting and press start.

Observe the dough as it kneads. After 5 to 10 minutes, if it appears dry and stiff or if your machine sounds as if it's straining to knead it, add more liquid 1 tablespoon at a time until dough forms a smooth, soft, pliable ball that is slightly tacky to the touch.

After the baking cycle ends, remove bread from pan, place on cake rack, and allow to cool 1 hour before slicing.

Nutrition:

Calories: 110 Cal

Carbohydrate: 19 g

Fat: 2 g

Protein: 4 g

5. Whole-Wheat Bread

Preparation Time: 1 hour 10 minutes

Cooking Time: 40 minutes

Servings: 1 loaf

Ingredients:

3/4 to 7/8 cup water

1 teaspoon Salt

3 tablespoon Butter or margarine

1 tablespoon Sugar

11/3 cups whole wheat flour

2/3 cups bread flour

3 tablespoon Instant potato flakes

11/2 teaspoon Active dry yeast optional:

2 tablespoon vital wheat gluten

Directions:

Using the least amount of the liquid indicated in the recipe, place all the Ingredients in the bread pan. Select medium crust then the whole wheat cycle. Press start.

After 5-10 minutes, observe the dough as it kneads, if you hear straining sounds in your machine or if the dough appears stiff and dry, add 1 tablespoon Liquid at a time until the dough becomes smooth, pliable, soft, and slightly tacky to the touch.

Remove the bread from the pan after baking. Place on rack and allow to cool for 1 hour before slicing.

Nutrition:

Calories: 60 Cal

Carbohydrate: 11 g

Fat: 1 g

Protein: 3 g

6. Awesome Golden Corn Bread

Preparation Time: 1 hour 10 minutes

Cooking Time: 50 minutes

Servings: 2 loaves

Ingredients:

1 cup buttermilk at 80 degrees F

2 whole eggs, at room temperature

¼ cup melted butter, cooled

1⅓ cups all-purpose flour

1 cup cornmeal

¼ cup sugar

1 tablespoon baking powder

1 teaspoon salt

Directions:

Add buttermilk, butter, and eggs to your bread machine, carefully following the manufacturer instructions.

Program the machine for *Quick/Rapid Bread* mode and press *START*.

While the wet ingredients are being mixed in the machine, take a small bowl and combine it in flour, cornmeal, sugar, baking powder, and salt.

After the first fast mix is done and the machine gives the signal, add dry ingredients.

Wait until the whole cycle completes.

Once the loaf is done, take the bucket out and let it cool for 5 minutes.

Gently shake the basket to remove the loaf and transfer to a cooling rack. Slice and serve!

Nutrition:

Calories: 158 Cal Fat: 5 g Carbohydrates:24 g Protein : 4 g

Fiber: 2 g

7. Hearty Oatmeal Bread

Preparation Time: 2 hours 10 minutes

Cooking Time: 50 minutes

Servings: 1 loaf

Ingredients:

¾ cup water at 80 degrees F

2 tablespoons melted butter, cooled

2 tablespoons sugar

1 teaspoon salt ¾ cup quick oats

1½ cups white bread flour

1 teaspoon instant yeast

Directions:

Add all of the ingredients to your bread machine, carefully following the

instructions of the manufacturer.

Set the program of your bread machine to Basic/White Bread and set

crust type to Medium.

Press START.

Wait until the cycle completes.

Once the loaf is ready, take the bucket out and let the loaf cool for 5

minutes.

Gently shake the bucket to remove the loaf.

Transfer to a cooling rack, slice, and serve.

Nutrition:

Calories: 149 Cal

Fat   : 4 g

Carbohydrates: 26 g

Protein : 4 g

Fiber: 1 g

8. Corn, Poppy Seeds and Sour Cream Bread

Preparation Time: 2 hours 40 minutes

Cooking Time: 50 minutes

Servings: 2 loaves

Ingredients:

3½ cups wheat flour

1¾ cups corn flour

5 ounces sour cream

2 tablespoons corn oil

2 teaspoons active dried yeast

2 teaspoons salt 16 ¼ ounces water

Poppy seeds for sprinkling

Directions:

Add 16¼ ounces of water and corn oil to the bread maker bucket.

Add flour, sour cream, sugar, and salt from different angles.

Make a groove in the flour and add yeast.

Set the program of your bread machine to Basic/White Bread and set crust type to Medium.

Press START.

Wait until the cycle completes.

Once the loaf is ready, take the bucket out and let the loaf cool for 5 minutes.

Gently shake the bucket to remove the loaf.

Moisten the surface with water and sprinkle with poppy seeds.

Transfer to a cooling rack, slice, and serve.

Nutrition:

Calories: 374 Cal

Fat: 10 g Carbohydrates:64 g

Protein: 9 g

Fiber: 1 g

9. Grampy's Special Bread

Preparation Time: 2 hours 30 minutes

Cooking Time: 40 minutes

Servings: 1 loaf

Ingredients:

1 1/4 cups skim milk

1 cup crispy rice cereal

3 cups bread flour 2 tablespoons honey

1 1/4 teaspoons salt

1 1/2 (.25 oz.) packages active dry yeast

2 tablespoons margarine

Directions:

Into the bread machine pan, add the ingredients according to the order given by manufacturer. Use Basic/White Bread setting and then press the Start button.

Nutrition:

Calories: 46 calories;

Total Carbohydrate: 6.5 g

Cholesterol: < 1 mg

Total Fat: 1.9 g

Protein: 1.4 g

Sodium: 292 mg

10.Butter Honey Wheat Bread

Preparation Time: 3 hours 5 minutes

Cooking Time: 15 minutes

Servings: 12

Ingredients:

1 cup water

2 tablespoons margarine

2 tablespoons honey

2 cups bread flour

1/2 cup whole wheat flour

1/3 cup dry milk powder

1 teaspoon salt 1 (.25 oz.) package active dry yeast

Directions:

Follow the order of putting the ingredients into the bread machine recommended by the manufacturer. Run the bread machine for large

loaf (1-1/2 lb.) on Wheat setting.

Nutrition:

Calories: 57 calories;

Total Carbohydrate: 8.5 g

Cholesterol: < 1 mg

Total Fat: 1.9 g

Protein: 2.1 g

Sodium: 234 mg

11. Buttermilk Wheat Bread

Preparation Time: 6 hours 8 minutes

Cooking Time: 15 minutes

Servings: 12

Ingredients:

1 1/2 cups buttermilk

1 1/2 tablespoons butter, melted

2 tablespoons white sugar

3/4 teaspoon salt 3 cups all-purpose flour

1/3 cup whole wheat flour

1 1/2 teaspoons active dry yeast

Directions:

In the bread machine pan, measure all ingredients in the order the

manufacturer recommended. Set the machine to the Basic White Bread setting. Start the machine. After a few minutes, add more buttermilk if the ingredients do not form a ball, or if it is too loose, put a handful of flour.

Nutrition:

Calories: 160 calories;

Total Carbohydrate: 30 g

Cholesterol: 5 mg

Total Fat: 2.1 g

Protein: 4.9 g

Sodium: 189 mg

Cheese Bread

12. Cheesy Chipotle Bread

Preparation Time: 2 hours

Cooking Time: 15 minutes

Servings: 8

Ingredients:

⅔ cup water, at 80°F to 90°F

1½ tablespoons sugar

1½ tablespoons powdered skim milk

¾ teaspoon salt

½ teaspoon chipotle chili powder

2 cups white bread flour

½ cup (2 ounces) shredded sharp Cheddar cheese

¾ teaspoon bread machine or instant yeast

Directions:

Place the ingredients in your bread machine as recommended by the manufacturer.

Program the machine for Basic/White bread, select light or medium crust, and press Start.

When the loaf is done, remove the bucket from the machine.

Let the loaf cool for 5 minutes.

Gently shake the bucket to remove the loaf, and turn it out onto a rack to cool..

Nutrition:

Calories: 139 calories;

Total Carbohydrate: 27 g otal Fat: 1g

Protein: 6 g Sodium: 245 mg

Fiber: 1 g

13.Cheddar Cheese Basil Bread

Preparation Time: 2 hours

Cooking Time: 15 minutes

Servings: 8

Ingredients:

⅔ cup milk, at 80°F to 90°F

2 teaspoons melted butter, cooled

2 teaspoons sugar

⅔ Teaspoon dried basil

½ cup (2 ounces) shredded sharp Cheddar cheese

½ teaspoon salt 2 cups white bread flour

1 teaspoon bread machine or active dry yeast

Directions:

Place the ingredients in your bread machine as recommended by the manufacturer.

Program the machine for Basic/White bread, select light or medium crust, and press Start.

When the loaf is done, remove the bucket from the machine.

Let the loaf cool for 5 minutes.

Gently shake the bucket to remove the loaf, and turn it out onto a rack to cool..

Nutrition:

Calories: 166 calories;

Total Carbohydrate: 26 g

Total Fat: 4g

Protein: 6 g

Sodium: 209 mg

Fiber: 1 g

14.Olive Cheese Bread

Preparation Time: 2 hours

Cooking Time: 15 minutes

Servings: 8

Ingredients:

⅔ Cup milk, at 80°F to 90°F

1 tablespoon melted butter, cooled

⅔ Teaspoon minced garlic

1 tablespoon sugar

⅔ Teaspoon salt

2 cups white bread flour

½ cup (2 ounces) shredded Swiss cheese

¾ teaspoon bread machine or instant yeast

¼ cup chopped black olives

Directions:

Place the ingredients in your bread machine as recommended by the manufacturer.

Program the machine for Basic/White bread, select light or medium crust, and press Start.

When the loaf is done, remove the bucket from the machine.

Let the loaf cool for 5 minutes.

Gently shake the bucket to remove the loaf, and turn it out onto a rack to cool..

Nutrition:

Calories: 175 calories;

Total Carbohydrate: 27 g

Total Fat: 5g Protein: 6 g

Sodium: 260 mg

Fiber: 1 g

15.Double Cheese Bread

Preparation Time: 2 hours

Cooking Time: 15 minutes

Servings: 8

Ingredients:

¾ cup plus 1 tablespoon milk, at 80°F to 90°F

2 teaspoons butter, melted and cooled

4 teaspoons sugar

⅔ teaspoon salt

⅓ teaspoon freshly ground black pepper

Pinch cayenne pepper

1 cup (4 ounces) shredded aged sharp Cheddar cheese

⅓ cup shredded or grated Parmesan cheese

2 cups white bread flour

¾ teaspoon bread machine or instant yeast

Directions:

Place the ingredients in your bread machine as recommended by the manufacturer.

Program the machine for Basic/White bread, select light or medium crust, and press Start.

When the loaf is done, remove the bucket from the machine.

Let the loaf cool for 5 minutes.

Gently shake the bucket to remove the loaf, and turn it out onto a rack to cool..

Nutrition:

Calories: 183 calories; Total Carbohydrate: 28 g

Total Fat: 4g Protein: 6 g

Sodium: 344 mg

Fiber: 1 g

16.Chile Cheese Bacon Bread

Preparation Time: 2 hours

Cooking Time: 15 minutes

Servings: 8

Ingredients:

⅓ Cup milk, at 80°F to 90°F

1 teaspoon melted butter, cooled

1 tablespoon honey

1 teaspoon salt

⅓ Cup chopped and drained green Chile

⅓ Cup grated Cheddar cheese

⅓ cup chopped cooked bacon

2 cups white bread flour

1⅓ teaspoons bread machine or instant yeast

Directions:

Place the ingredients in your bread machine as recommended by the manufacturer.

Program the machine for Basic/White bread, select light or medium crust, and press Start.

When the loaf is done, remove the bucket from the machine.

Let the loaf cool for 5 minutes.

Gently shake the bucket to remove the loaf, and turn it out onto a rack to cool..

Nutrition:

Calories: 174 calories;

Total Carbohydrate: 404 g

Total Fat: 4 g Protein: 6 g

Sodium: 1 mg

Fiber: 1 g

17.Italian Parmesan Bread

Preparation Time: 2 hours

Cooking Time: 15 minutes

Servings: 8

Ingredients:

¾ cup water, at 80°F to 90°F

2 tablespoons melted butter, cooled

2 teaspoons sugar ⅔ teaspoon salt

1⅓ teaspoons chopped fresh basil

2⅔ tablespoons grated Parmesan cheese

2⅓ cups white bread flour 1 teaspoon bread machine or instant yeast

Directions:

Place the ingredients in your bread machine as recommended by the

manufacturer.

Program the machine for Basic/White bread, select light or medium crust, and press Start.

When the loaf is done, remove the bucket from the machine.

Let the loaf cool for 5 minutes.

Gently shake the bucket to remove the loaf, and turn it out onto a rack to cool..

Nutrition:

Calories: 171 calories;

Total Carbohydrate: 29 g

Total Fat: 4 g

Protein: 5 g

Sodium: 237 mg

Fiber: 1 g

18.Feta Oregano Bread

Preparation Time: 2 hours

Cooking Time: 15 minutes

Servings: 8

Ingredients:

⅔ Cup milk, at 80°F to 90°F

2 teaspoons melted butter, cooled

2 teaspoons sugar

⅔ Teaspoon salt

2 teaspoons dried oregano

2 cups white bread flour

1½ teaspoons bread machine or instant yeast

⅔ cup (2½ ounces) crumbled feta cheese

Directions:

Place the ingredients in your bread machine as recommended by the manufacturer.

Program the machine for Basic/White bread, select light or medium crust, and press Start.

When the loaf is done, remove the bucket from the machine.

Let the loaf cool for 5 minutes.

Gently shake the bucket to remove the loaf, and turn it out onto a rack to cool..

Nutrition:

Calories: 164 calories;

Total Carbohydrate: 27 g

Total Fat: 4 g

Protein: 5 g

Sodium: 316 mg

Fiber: 2 g

Fruit Breads

19.Peaches and Cream Bread

Preparation Time: 2 hours

Cooking Time: 15 minutes **Servings:** 8

Ingredients:

½ cup canned peaches, drained and chopped

¼ cup heavy whipping cream, at 80°F to 90°F

1 egg, at room temperature

¾ tablespoon melted butter, cooled

1½ tablespoons sugar

¾ teaspoon salt

¼ teaspoon ground cinnamon

⅛ teaspoon ground nutmeg

¼ cup whole-wheat flour

1¾ cups white bread flour

¾ teaspoons bread machine or instant yeast

Directions:

Place the ingredients in your bread machine as recommended by the

manufacturer.

Program the machine for Basic/White bread, select light or medium

crust, and press Start.

When the loaf is done, remove the bucket from the machine.

Let the loaf cool for 5 minutes.

Gently shake the bucket to remove the loaf, and turn it out onto a rack

to cool..

Nutrition:

Calories: 153 calories; Total Carbohydrate: 27 g Total Fat: 4 g

Protein: 5 g Sodium: 208 mg iber: 1 g

20. Warm Spiced Pumpkin Bread

Preparation Time: 2 hours

Cooking Time: 15 minutes

Servings: 12- 16

Ingredients:

Butter for greasing the bucket

1½ cups pumpkin purée

3 eggs, at room temperature

⅓ cup melted butter, cooled

1 cup sugar

3 cups all-purpose flour

1½ teaspoons baking powder

¾ teaspoon ground cinnamon

½ teaspoon baking soda

¼ teaspoon ground nutmeg

¼ teaspoon ground ginger

¼ teaspoon salt

Pinch ground cloves

Directions:

Lightly grease the bread bucket with butter.

Add the pumpkin, eggs, butter, and sugar.

Program the machine for Quick/Rapid bread and press Start.

Let the wet ingredients be mixed by the paddles until the first fast mixing

cycle is finished, about 10 minutes into the cycle.

Stir together the flour, baking powder, cinnamon, baking soda, nutmeg,

ginger, salt, and cloves until well blended.

Add the dry ingredients to the bucket when the second fast mixing cycle

starts.

When the loaf is done, remove the bucket from the machine.

Let the loaf cool for 5 minutes.

Gently shake the bucket to remove the loaf, and turn it out onto a rack to cool.

Nutrition:

Calories: 251 calories;

Total Carbohydrate: 43 g

Total Fat: 7 g

Protein: 5 g

Sodium: 159 mg

Fiber: 2 g

21.Pure Peach Bread

Preparation Time: 2 hours

Cooking Time: 15 minutes

Servings: 12

Ingredients:

¾ cup peaches, chopped

⅓ cup heavy whipping cream

1 egg 1 tablespoon butter, melted at room temperature

⅓ teaspoon ground cinnamon

⅛ teaspoon ground nutmeg

2 ¼ tablespoons sugar

1 ⅛ teaspoons salt

⅓ cup whole-wheat flour

2 ⅔ cups white bread flour

1 ⅛ teaspoons instant or bread machine yeast

Directions:

Take 1 ½ pound size loaf pan and first add the liquid ingredients and then add the dry ingredients.

Place the loaf pan in the machine and close its top lid.

For selecting a bread cycle, press "Basic Bread/White Bread/Regular Bread" and for selecting a crust type, press "Light" or "Medium".

Start the machine and it will start preparing the bread.

After the bread loaf is completed, open the lid and take out the loaf pan.

Allow the pan to cool down for 10-15 minutes on a wire rack. Gently shake the pan and remove the bread loaf.

Make slices and serve.

Nutrition:

Calories: 51 calories; Total Carbohydrate: 12 g Cholesterol: 0 g

Total Fat: 0.3 g Protein: 1.20 g Fiber: 2 g

22.   Date Delight Bread

Preparation Time: 2 hours

Cooking Time: 15 minutes

Servings: 12

Ingredients:

¾ cup water, lukewarm

½ cup milk, lukewarm

2 tablespoons butter, melted at room temperature

¼ cup honey

3 tablespoons molasses

1 tablespoon sugar

2 ¼ cups whole-wheat flour

1 ¼ cups white bread flour

2 tablespoons skim milk powder

1 teaspoon salt

1 tablespoon unsweetened cocoa powder

1 ½ teaspoons instant or bread machine yeast

¾ cup chopped dates

Directions:

Take 1 ½ pound size loaf pan and first add the liquid ingredients and then add the dry ingredients. (Do not add the dates as of now.)

Place the loaf pan in the machine and close its top lid.

Plug the bread machine into power socket. For selecting a bread cycle, press "Basic Bread/White Bread/Regular Bread" or "Fruit/Nut Bread" and for selecting a crust type, press "Light" or "Medium".

Start the machine and it will start preparing the bread. When machine beeps or signals, add the dates.

After the bread loaf is completed, open the lid and take out the loaf pan.

Allow the pan to cool down for 10-15 minutes on a wire rack. Gently shake the pan and remove the bread loaf.

Make slices and serve.

Nutrition:

Calories: 220 calories;

Total Carbohydrate: 52 g

Cholesterol: 0 g

Total Fat: 5 g

Protein: 4 g

23. Blueberry Honey Bread

Preparation Time: 2 hours

Cooking Time: 15 minutes

Servings: 12

Ingredients:

¾ cup milk, lukewarm

1 egg, at room temperature

2 ¼ tablespoons butter, melted at room temperature

1 ½ tablespoons honey

½ cup rolled oats 2 ⅓ cups white bread flour

1 ⅛ teaspoons salt 1 ½ teaspoons instant or bread machine yeast

½ cup dried blueberries

Directions:

Take 1 ½ pound size loaf pan and first add the liquid ingredients and then add the dry ingredients. (Do not add the blueberries as of now.)

Place the loaf pan in the machine and close its top lid.

Plug the bread machine into power socket. For selecting a bread cycle, press "Basic Bread/White Bread/Regular Bread" or "Fruit/Nut Bread" and for selecting a crust type, press "Light" or "Medium".

Start the machine and it will start preparing the bread. When machine beeps or signals, add the blueberries.

After the bread loaf is completed, open the lid and take out the loaf pan.

Allow the pan to cool down for 10-15 minutes on a wire rack. Gently shake the pan and remove the bread loaf.

Make slices and serve.

Nutrition:

Calories: 180 calories;

Total Carbohydrate: 250 g

Total Fat: 3 g

Protein: 9 g

Vegetable Breads

24.   Spinach Bread

Preparation Time: 2 hours 20 minutes

Cooking Time: 40 minutes

Servings: 1 loaf

Ingredients:

1 cup water

1 tablespoon vegetable oil

1/2 cup frozen chopped spinach, thawed and drained

3 cups all-purpose flour

1/2 cup shredded Cheddar cheese

1 teaspoon salt

1 tablespoon white sugar

1/2 teaspoon ground black pepper

2 1/2 teaspoons active dry yeast

Directions:

In the pan of bread machine, put all ingredients according to the suggested order of manufacture. Set white bread cycle.

Nutrition:

Calories: 121 calories;

Total Carbohydrate: 20.5 g

Cholesterol: 4 mg

Total Fat: 2.5 g

Protein: 4 g

Sodium: 184 mg

25. Curd Bread

Preparation Time: 4 hours

Cooking Time: 15 minutes **Servings:** 12

Ingredients:

¾ cup lukewarm water 3 2/3 cups wheat bread machine flour

¾ cup cottage cheese 2 Tablespoon softened butter

2 Tablespoon white sugar

1½ teaspoon sea salt

1½ Tablespoon sesame seeds

2 Tablespoon dried onions

1¼ teaspoon bread machine yeast

Directions:

Place all the dry and liquid ingredients in the pan and follow the instructions for your bread machine.

Pay particular attention to measuring the ingredients. Use a measuring cup, measuring spoon, and kitchen scales to do so.

Set the baking program to BASIC and the crust type to MEDIUM.

If the dough is too dense or too wet, adjust the amount of flour and liquid in the recipe.

When the program has ended, take the pan out of the bread machine and let cool for 5 minutes.

Shake the loaf out of the pan. If necessary, use a spatula.

Wrap the bread with a kitchen towel and set it aside for an hour. Otherwise, you can cool it on a wire rack.

Nutrition:

Calories: 277 calories;

Total Carbohydrate: 48.4 g Cholesterol: 9 g

Total Fat: 4.7g Protein: 9.4 g

Sodium: 547 mg Sugar: 3.3 g

26. Curvy Carrot Bread

Preparation Time: 2 hours

Cooking Time: 15 minutes

Servings: 12

Ingredients:

¾ cup milk, lukewarm

3 tablespoons butter, melted at room temperature

1 tablespoon honey ¾ teaspoon ground nutmeg

½ teaspoon salt 1 ½ cups shredded carrot

3 cups white bread flour

2 ¼ teaspoons bread machine or active dry yeast

Directions:

Take 1 ½ pound size loaf pan and first add the liquid ingredients and then add the dry ingredients.

Place the loaf pan in the machine and close its top lid.

Plug the bread machine into power socket. For selecting a bread cycle, press "Quick Bread/Rapid Bread" and for selecting a crust type, press "Light" or "Medium".

Start the machine and it will start preparing the bread.

After the bread loaf is completed, open the lid and take out the loaf pan.

Allow the pan to cool down for 10-15 minutes on a wire rack. Gently shake the pan and remove the bread loaf.

Make slices and serve.

Nutrition:

Calories: 142 calories;

Total Carbohydrate: 32.2 g

Cholesterol: 0 g

Total Fat: 0.8 g

Protein: 2.33 g

27.   Potato Rosemary Bread

Preparation Time: 3 hours

Cooking Time: 30 minutes

Servings: 20

Ingredients:

4 cups bread flour, sifted 1 tablespoon white sugar

1 tablespoon sunflower oil 1½ teaspoons salt 1½ cups lukewarm water

1 teaspoon active dry yeast 1 cup potatoes, mashed

2 teaspoons crushed rosemary

Directions:

Prepare all of the ingredients for your bread and measuring means (a

cup, a spoon, kitchen scales).

Carefully measure the ingredients into the pan, except the potato and

rosemary.

Place all of the ingredients into the bread bucket in the right order, following the manual for your bread machine.

Close the cover.

Select the program of your bread machine to BREAD with FILLINGS and choose the crust color to MEDIUM.

Press START.

After the signal, put the mashed potato and rosemary to the dough.

Wait until the program completes.

When done, take the bucket out and let it cool for 5-10 minutes.

Shake the loaf from the pan and let cool for 30 minutes on a cooling rack.

Slice, serve and enjoy the taste of fragrant homemade bread.

Nutrition:

Calories: 106 calories; Total Carbohydrate: 21 g Total Fat: 1 g

Protein: 2.9 g Sodium: 641 mg Fiber: 1 g

Sugar: 0.8 g

28. Beetroot Prune Bread

Preparation Time: 3 hours

Cooking Time: 30 minutes

Servings: 20

Ingredients:

1½ cups lukewarm beet broth 5¼ cups all-purpose flour

1 cup beet puree 1 cup prunes, chopped

4 tablespoons extra virgin olive oil

2 tablespoons dry cream 1 tablespoon brown sugar

2 teaspoons active dry yeast 1 tablespoon whole milk

2 teaspoons sea salt

Directions:

Prepare all of the ingredients for your bread and measuring means (a

cup, a spoon, kitchen scales).

Carefully measure the ingredients into the pan, except the prunes.

Place all of the ingredients into the bread bucket in the right order, following the manual for your bread machine.

Close the cover.

Select the program of your bread machine to BASIC and choose the crust color to MEDIUM. Press START. After the signal, put the prunes to the dough.

Wait until the program completes.

When done, take the bucket out and let it cool for 5-10 minutes.

Shake the loaf from the pan and let cool for 30 minutes on a cooling rack.

Slice, serve and enjoy the taste of fragrant homemade bread.

Nutrition:

Calories: 443 calories; Total Carbohydrate: 81.1 g

Total Fat: 8.2 g Protein: 9.9 g Sodium: 604 mg

Fiber: 4.4 g Sugar: 11.7 g

Sourdough Breads

29. Crusty Sourdough Bread

Preparation Time: 15 minutes ; 1 week (Starter)

Cooking Time: 3 hours **Servings:** 1 loaf

Ingredients:

1/2 cup water 3 cups bread flour 2 tablespoons sugar

1 ½ teaspoon salt 1 teaspoon bread machine or quick active dry yeast

Directions:

Measure 1 cup of starter and remaining bread ingredients, add to bread

machine pan.

Nutrition: Calories: 165 calories; Total Carbohydrate: 37 g Total Fat: 0 g

Protein: 5 g Sodium: 300 mg Fiber: 1 g

30. Honey Sourdough Bread

Preparation Time: 15 minutes ; 1 week (Starter)

Cooking Time: 3 hours

Servings: 1 loaf

Ingredients:

2/3 cup sourdough starter

1/2 cup water

1 tablespoon vegetable oil

2 tablespoons honey

1/2 teaspoon salt

1/2 cup high protein wheat flour

2 cups bread flour

1 teaspoon active dry yeast

Directions:

Measure 1 cup of starter and remaining bread ingredients, add to bread machine pan.

Choose basic/white bread cycle with medium or light crust color.

Nutrition:

Calories: 175 calories;

Total Carbohydrate: 33 g

Total Fat: 0.3 g

Protein: 5.6 g

Sodium: 121 mg

Fiber: 1.9 g

31.Multigrain Sourdough Bread

Preparation Time: 15 minutes ; 1 week (Starter)

Cooking Time: 3 hours

Servings: 1 loaf

Ingredients:

2 cups sourdough starter

2 tablespoons butter or 2 tablespoons olive oil

1/2 cup milk

1 teaspoon salt 1/4 cup honey 1/2 cup sunflower seeds

1/2 cup millet or 1/2 cup amaranth or 1/2 cup quinoa

3 1/2 cups multi-grain flour

Directions:

Add ingredients to bread machine pan.

Choose dough cycle.

Conventional Oven:

When cycle is complete, remove dough and place on lightly floured surface and shape into loaf.

Place in greased loaf pan, cover, and rise until bread is a couple inches above the edge.

Bake at 375 degrees for 40 to 50 minutes.

Nutrition:

Calories: 110 calories;

Total Carbohydrate: 13.5 g

Total Fat: 1.8 g

Protein: 2.7 g

Sodium: 213 mg

Fiber: 1.4 g

32. Olive and Garlic Sourdough Bread

Preparation Time: 15 minutes ; 1 week (Starter)

Cooking Time: 3 hours

Servings: 1 loaf

Ingredients:

2 cups sourdough starter

3 cups flour

2 tablespoons olive oil

2 tablespoons sugar

2 teaspoon salt

1/2 cup chopped black olives

6 cloves chopped garlic

Directions:

Add starter and bread ingredients to bread machine pan.

Choose dough cycle.

Conventional Oven:

Preheat oven to 350 degrees.

When cycle is complete, if dough is sticky add more flour.

Shape dough onto baking sheet or put into loaf pan

Bake for 35- 45 minutes until golden.

Cool before slicing.

Nutrition:

Calories: 150 calories;

Total Carbohydrate: 26.5 g

Total Fat: 0.5 g

Protein: 3.4 g

Sodium: 267 mg

Fiber: 1.1 g

33. Czech Sourdough Bread

Preparation Time: 15 minutes ; 1 week (Starter)

Cooking Time: 3 hours

Servings: 1 loaf

Ingredients:

1 cup non-dairy milk

1 tablespoon salt

1 tablespoon honey

1 cup sourdough starter

1 1/2 cups rye flour

1 cup bread flour

3/4 cup wheat flour

1/2 cup grated half-baked potato

5 tablespoons wheat gluten

2 teaspoons caraway seeds

Directions:

Add ingredients to bread machine pan.

Choose the dough cycle.

The dough will need to rise, up to 24 hours, in the bread machine until

doubles in size.

After rising, bake in bread machine for one hour.

Nutrition:

Calories: 198 calories;

Total Carbohydrate: 39.9 g

Total Fat: 0.8 g

Protein: 6.5 g

Sodium: 888 mg

Fiber: 4.3 g

34. French Sourdough Bread

Preparation Time: 15 minutes ; 1 week (Starter)

Cooking Time: 3 hours

Servings: 2 loaf

Ingredients:

2 cups sourdough starter 1 teaspoon salt 1/2 cup water

4 cups white bread flour 2 tablespoons white cornmeal

Directions:

Add ingredients to bread machine pan, saving cornmeal for later.

Choose dough cycle.

Conventional Oven:

Preheat oven to 375 degrees.

At end of dough cycle, turn dough out onto a floured surface.

Add flour if dough is sticky.

Divide dough into 2 portions and flatten into an oval shape 1 ½ inch thick.

Fold ovals in half lengthwise and pinch seams to elongate.

Sprinkle cornmeal onto baking sheet and place the loaves seam side down.

Cover and let rise in until about doubled.

Place a shallow pan of hot water on the lower shelf of the oven;

Use a knife to make shallow, diagonal slashes in tops of loaves

Place the loaves in the oven and spray with fine water mister. Spray the oven walls as well.

Repeat spraying 3 times at one minute intervals.

Remove pan of water after 15 minutes of baking

Fully bake for 30 to 40 minutes or until golden brown.

Nutrition:

Calories: 937 calories; Total Carbohydrate: 196 g Total Fat: 0.4 g

Protein: 26.5 g Sodium: 1172 mg Fiber: 7.3 g

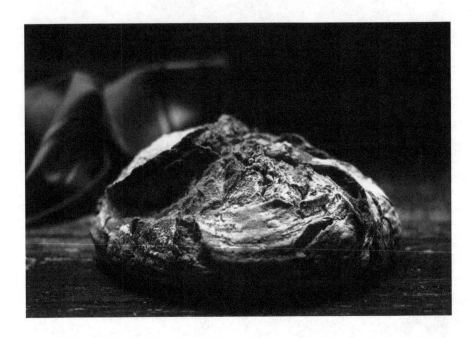

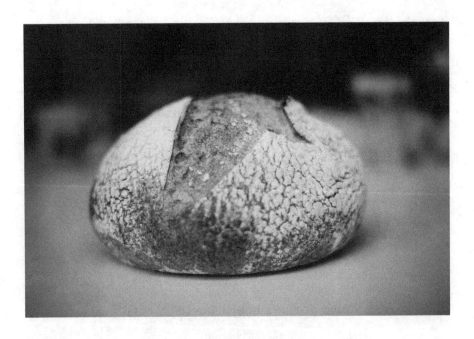

Sweet Breads

35.   Peanut Butter Bread

Preparation Time: 10 minutes

Cooking Time: 3 hours

Servings: 1 loaf

Ingredients:

1 1/4 Cups water

1/2 cup Peanut butter - creamy or chunky

1 ½ cups whole wheat flour

3 tablespoons Gluten flour

1 ½ cups bread flour

1/4 cup Brown sugar

1/2 teaspoon Salt -

2 ¼ teaspoons Active dry yeast

Directions:

Add all the ingredients into pan.

Choose whole wheat bread setting, large loaf.

Nutrition:

Calories: 82 calories;

Total Carbohydrate: 13 g

Cholesterol: 13 mg

Total Fat: 2.2 g

Protein: 2.5 g

Sodium: 280 mg

Fiber: 1 g

36.   Sweet Pineapples Bread

Preparation Time: 2 hours

Cooking Time: 40 minutes

Servings: 5

Ingredients:

8 oz dried pineapples

4 oz raisins

5 oz wheat flour

3 eggs

3 teaspoon baking powder

8 oz brown sugar 2 oz sugar Vanilla

Directions:

Place the raisins into the warm water and leave for 20 minutes.

In a bowl, combine the sifted wheat flour, baking powder, brown sugar and vanilla.

Add the raisins and pineapples and mix well.

Whisk the eggs with the sugar until they have a smooth and creamy consistency.

Combine the eggs mixture with the flour and dried fruits mixture.

Pour the dough into the bread machine, close the lid and turn the bread machine on the basic/white bread program.

Bake the bread until the medium crust and after the bread is ready take it out and leave for 1 hour covered with the towel and only then you can slice the bread.

Nutrition:

Calories: 144 calories;

Total Carbohydrate: 18 g

Total Fat: 9 g

Protein: 6 g

37.   Sweet Coconut Bread

Preparation Time: 2 hours

Cooking Time: 40 minutes

Servings: 6

Ingredients:

8 oz shredded coconut

4 oz walnuts, ground

5 oz wheat flour

3 oz coconut butter

3 eggs

3 teaspoon baking powder

6 oz brown sugar Vanilla

Directions:

Whisk the eggs until they have a smooth and creamy consistency.

Combine the coconut butter with the brown sugar and vanilla and mix well, adding the eggs.

Combine the sifted wheat flour with the baking powder and eggs mixture and mix well until they have a smooth consistency.

Combine the dough with the shredded coconut and walnuts and then mix well.

Pour the dough into the bread machine, close the lid and turn the bread machine on the basic/white bread program.

Bake the bread until the medium crust and after the bread is ready take it out and leave for 1 hour covered with the towel and only then you can slice the bread.

Nutrition:

Calories: 164 calories; Total Carbohydrate: 12 g Total Fat: 8 g

Protein: 7 g

Soft Breads, Vegan White

Bread, French Bread, Pumpkin

Bread ecc.

38. Honey Sandwich Bread

Preparation Time: 5 minutes

Cooking Time: 55 minutes

Servings: 1 loaf

Ingredients:

¼ c honey

½ teaspoon salt

1 ½ lukewarm water,

2 ¼ teaspoons active dry yeast

2 tablespoons olive oil

4 ¼ cups whole-wheat flour

Directions:

Place your ingredients onto the bread machine pan.

Create a dip well unto the dry ingredients and place your wet ingredients

here.

Choose the whole wheat cycle and start.

Wait and serve. Enjoy!

Nutrition:

Calories: 86 Cal

Fat   : 2.5 g

Carbohydrates: 4.8 g

Protein : 1 g

39.   Honey Buttermilk Bread

Preparation Time: 10 minutes

Cooking Time: 2 hours

Servings: 1 loaf

Ingredients:

1 1/2 teaspoons salt

1/2 c water

2 teaspoons yeast

3 c bread flour

3 tablespoons honey

3 teaspoons butter 3/4 c buttermilk

Directions:

Place all ingredients in the bread machine pan.

Select the dough cycle.

Mold it into a loaf and lay it on a baking pan lined with grease parchment.

Glaze with egg wash. You can also top it with sesame seeds if preferred.

Pop it into the oven for about 30 mins at a temp of 190°C (375°F).

Enjoy!

Nutrition:

Calories: 92 Cal

Fat: 5.4 g

Carbohydrates: 2.4 g

Protein: 1 g

Keto Breads

40. Lemon Poppy Seed Bread

Preparation Time: 10 minutes

Cooking Time: 4 hours

Servings: 6

Ingredients:

3 eggs, pasteurized

1 ½ tablespoons butter, grass-fed, unsalted, melted

1 ½ tablespoons lemon juice

1 lemon, zested

1 ½ cups / 150 grams almond flour

¼ cup / 50 grams erythritol sweetener

¼ teaspoon baking powder

1 tablespoon poppy seeds

Directions:

Gather all the ingredients for the bread and plug in the bread machine having the capacity of 1 pound of bread recipe.

Take a large bowl, crack eggs in it and then beat in butter, lemon juice, and lemon zest until combined.

Take a separate large bowl, add flour in it and then stir in sweetener, baking powder, and poppy seeds until mixed.

Add egg mixture into the bread bucket, top with flour mixture, shut the lid, select the "basic/white" cycle or "low-carb" setting and then press the up/down arrow button to adjust baking time according to your bread machine; it will take 3 to 4 hours.

Then press the crust button to select light crust if available, and press the "start/stop" button to switch on the bread machine.

When the bread machine beeps, open the lid, then take out the bread basket and lift out the bread.

Let bread cool on a wire rack for 1 hour, then cut it into six slices and

serve.

Nutrition:

Calories: 201 Cal

Fat: 17.5 g

Carbohydrates: 5.8 g

Protein : 8.2 g

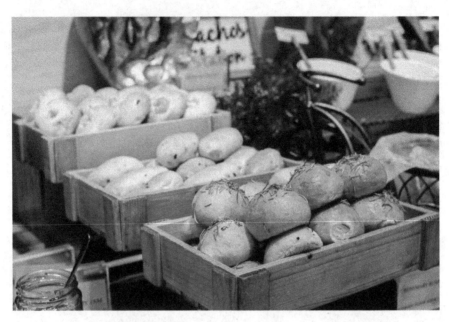

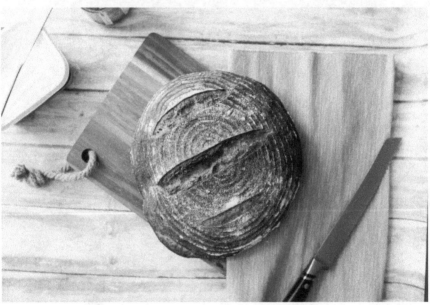

Conclusion

Depending on what kind of home baker you are, bread is either a must-know rite of passage, or an intimidating goal you haven't quite worked up the courage to try. This is because bread is a labor-intensive food where slight mistakes can have a big impact on the final result. Most of us rely on store-bought bread, but once you've tasted homemade bread, it's tempting to make your own as often as possible. A bread machine makes the process easier.

Making a loaf of bread feels like a major accomplishment. Why? There are a lot of steps. Mixing, kneading, proofing, resting, shaping, and finally baking.

You know how to make bread by hand, so how does the bread-making machine do it? A bread machine is basically a small, electric oven. It fits one large bread tin with a special axle connected to the electric motor. A metal paddle connects to the axle, and this is what kneads the dough. If you were making the bread in a mixer, you would probably use a dough hook, and in some instructions, you'll see the bread machine's kneading part referred as a hook or "blades."

The first thing you do is take out the tin and add the bread dough you made in Step 1. Bread machines can make any kind of bread, whether it's made from normal white flour, whole wheat, etc. Pop this tin unto the axle and program by selecting the type of bread, which includes options like basic, whole-wheat, multigrain, and so on. There are even cycles specifically for sweet breads; breads with nuts, seeds, and raisins; gluten-free; and bagels. Many models also let you cook jam.

You'll probably see a "dough" mode option, too. You would use that one for pizza. The machine doesn't actually cook anything; it just kneads and then you take out the pizza dough and bake it in your normal oven. If you aren't making pizza dough, the next selections you'll make are the loaf size and crust type. Once those are chosen, press the "timer" button. Based on your other selections, a time will show up and all you have to do is push "start."

After kneading and before the machine begins baking, many people will remove the dough so they can take out the kneading paddles, since they often make an indent in the finished bread. The paddles should simply pop out or you can buy a special hook that makes the removal easier. Now you can return the bread to the machine. The lid is closed during the baking process. If it's a glass lid, you can actually see what's going on. You'll hear the paddle spinning on the motor, kneading the dough. It lies still for the rising stage, and then starts again for more kneading if necessary. The motor is also off for the proving stage. Next, the heating element switches on, and steam rises from the exhaust vent as the bread bakes. The whole process usually takes a few hours.

There's a lot of work involved in making bread by hand. When you use a machine, that machine does a lot of the busy stuff for you. You just add your dough and the bread maker starts doing its thing, giving you time to do other chores or sit back and relax. As a note, not all bread makers are completely automatic, so if you want this benefit, you'll probably have to pay a bit more money. It's worth it for a lot of people, though.

Bread machines are indeed easy to use. If you can use a crockpot or a microwave, you can use a bread machine. Cycles and other settings like loaf size and color are always clearly marked, and once you do a quick read of your instruction manual, you'll be ready to go. Recipes written for bread makers are also very clear about what settings you need to select, so as long as you follow them, your bread will turn out the way you want.